CANNABIS EXTRACTS FOR BEGINNERS

Learn how to make your own extracts, from hash to wax

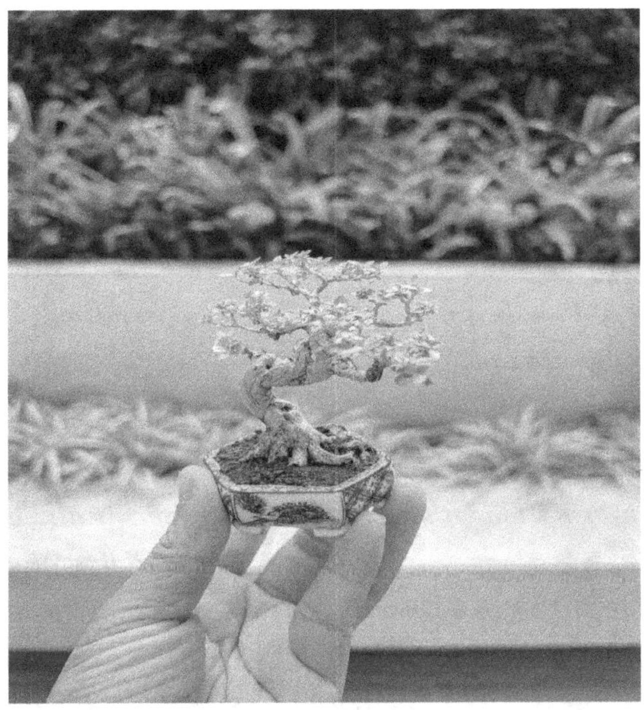

Mia Olivia

Copyright © 2023 by Mia Olivia

Disclaimer

This book is designed to provide condensed information. It's not intended to reprint all the information that is otherwise available, but instead to complement, amplify and supplement other texts. You are urged to read all available materials, learn as much as possible and tailor the information to your individual needs.

The purpose of this book is to educate.

TABLE OF CONTENTS

FOREWORD

"Welcome to the world of cannabis extracts! Whether you're an experienced user or just starting to explore the benefits of this versatile plant, this book is for you. Cannabis extracts have become an increasingly popular way to consume cannabis, but they can also be intimidating for beginners. In this book, you'll find a comprehensive guide to everything you need to know about cannabis extracts, from the basics of what they are to how they're made, how they're used, and how to make your own.

Whether you're interested in vaping, dabbing, or cooking with extracts, this book will provide you with the knowledge and tools you need to make informed decisions about your cannabis consumption. And if you're interested in trying your hand at making your own extracts, you'll find clear and helpful instructions on how to do so safely and effectively.

Don't let lack of knowledge hold you back from enjoying the benefits of cannabis extracts. With the information and guidance in this book, you can explore the world of cannabis extracts and discover new ways to enhance your experience.

"As a passionate advocate for cannabis and its many uses, I am excited to share this book with you. If you're new to the world of cannabis extracts, you have come to the right place. In these pages, you will find everything you need to know about this rapidly developing and increasingly popular form of cannabis consumption. From the basics of what extracts are and how they're made, to the various methods of consumption and the safety considerations that come with them, this book is a comprehensive guide to everything you need to know about cannabis extracts. Whether you're interested in vaping, dabbing, or cooking with extracts, you'll find that there are countless options to explore. And if you're interested in making your own extracts, you'll find clear and helpful instructions on how to do so safely and effectively. But more important than just providing information, this book is also a celebration of the unique culture and community that has developed around cannabis and its many uses. It is my hope that, by reading this book, you will gain a better understanding of what cannabis can offer, and become part of a community that values knowledge, collaboration, and empowerment.

The world of cannabis extracts is constantly changing and evolving, and it's exciting to be a part of that evolution. I hope that this book will help you to navigate this complex and sometimes confusing landscape, and empower you to make informed decisions about your cannabis consumption. If you're looking for a comprehensive guide to cannabis extracts that is both informative and accessible, then look no further.

Whether you're an experienced user or just starting out on your cannabis journey, you'll find that there is a wealth of knowledge and insight to be gained from these pages. I hope you'll enjoy your time with this book as much as I enjoyed creating it.

ACKNOWLEDGMENT

"The creation of this book would not have been possible without the support and guidance of many people.

First and foremost, I want to express my deep gratitude to all those who have contributed their knowledge and expertise to the world of cannabis extracts. Your passion and dedication to the industry have been paramount in shaping the landscape we know today.

Secondly, I would like to thank my family and friends for their unwavering support throughout this journey. Your love and encouragement have helped me to stay focused and motivated, and I am endlessly grateful for your presence in my life.

Finally, I want to acknowledge those who have contributed to the creation of this book in a more direct way. Your input and expertise have been invaluable, and I couldn't have done it without you. Your time and dedication to this project are greatly appreciated, and I am honored to be associated with such incredible individuals.

It is my hope that this book will serve as a valuable resource for anyone interested in the world of cannabis extracts. Whether you are a seasoned professional or a beginner looking to explore this exciting industry, I trust that you will find something of value in these pages. Thank you for taking the time to read this book, and I wish you all the best on your own cannabis extraction journey.

1

HISTORY AND CULTURE OF CANNABIS

Cannabis, also known as marijuana or weed, is a psychoactive drug that has been used by humans for thousands of years. While the exact origins of cannabis are unknown, it is thought to have first been cultivated and used for its psychoactive and medicinal properties in ancient Asia, particularly in the areas of modern-day India and China.

In ancient India, cannabis was used as a medicinal agent to treat a variety of ailments, including insomnia, pain, and inflammation. In ancient China, cannabis was commonly used as a treatment for various ailments, including stomachaches, headaches, and skin problems.

Cannabis was introduced to the West in the late 19th century, when it was brought by travelers from Asia. It was initially used as a medicinal herb, but as the knowledge of its psychoactive properties became more widespread, it began to be used recreationally as well.

Today, cannabis is the most widely used illegal drug in the world, with millions of people using it for both medicinal and recreational purposes. While its exact legalization status varies by country and jurisdiction, more and more countries are allowing for the use of cannabis for medical purposes, and some have even legalized its use for recreational purposes.

In addition to its use as a psychoactive substance, cannabis has also been used for a variety of other purposes throughout history. For example, it has been used in the production of textiles, rope, and paper, and as an ingredient in foods and beverages.

Despite the long and colorful history of cannabis, it has also been the subject of controversy and debate. Many countries have strict laws controlling its production, sale, and use, and there are ongoing discussions about the drug's potential benefits and harms.

Despite these controversies, cannabis remains an important cultural and historical phenomenon, and its impact on the world and society is sure to continue to be felt for years to come.

Cannabis has played a significant role in human history, with evidence of its use dating back thousands of years. It was originally used for medicinal purposes, but it gradually became popular as a recreational drug as well. Today, it is the most widely used illegal drug in the world. Its history, culture, and impact on society continue to be a topic of interest and study.

2

THE SCIENCE BEHIND CANNABIS EXTRACTION

Cannabis extraction is a process used to extract the psychoactive and therapeutic compounds from the cannabis plant. The active components of the plant, known as cannabinoids, are found mainly in a sticky, resinous substance known as trichomes, which are present on the surface of the plant. The most common cannabinoids in cannabis are THC (tetrahydrocannabinol) and CBD (cannabidiol), although there are many others that are present in smaller amounts.

To extract these cannabinoids, cannabis must first be grown and processed into some form that can be used for extraction. This typically involves drying and curing the cannabis to remove excess moisture and preserve the quality and potency of the trichomes. The resulting material is then processed using one of several different methods, including:

1. Solvent extraction: In this method, cannabis is processed using a solvent such as butane, ethanol, or hexane. This dissolves the cannabinoids into the solvent, which can then be separated from the plant material and concentrated into

an extract. This method is often used to create marijuana extracts such as hash oil and butane hash oil.

2. Non-solvent extraction: In this method, the cannabinoids are separated from the plant material using techniques such as ice water extraction, CO_2 extraction, or press extraction. These methods use no solvent and are considered to be safer and more efficient than solvent extraction.

3. Terpene extraction: Terpenes are the aromatic compounds present in cannabis that give the plant its unique scent. Terpene extraction can be done using methods such as steam distillation or CO_2 extraction, and the resulting terpene extract can be used to enhance the aroma and flavor of cannabis products.

Once the cannabinoids have been extracted, they can be purified and concentrated to create different types of cannabis products, including:

1. Dry sift hash: This is a refined form of hash that is produced by separating the trichomes from the plant material using screens or sifting techniques. The resulting hash is a soft, oily substance that can be smoked or used in cooking.

2. Rosin: Rosin is a solventless concentrate that is separated from the plant materials using high pressure and heat. It is a golden, oily substance that is known for its pure, unadulterated flavor.

It's important to note that the process of cannabis extraction is a complex and high regulated industry and the safety of the final product depends on efficient techniques.

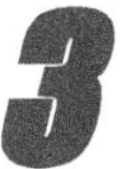

TOOLS AND MATERIALS NEEDED FOR CANNABIS EXTRACTION

Cannabis extraction involves using a variety of tools and materials to separate the trichomes from the plant material and extract the cannabinoids. Here is a list of some common tools and materials used for cannabis extraction:

1. **Cannabis Flower:** This is the starting material for cannabis extraction and is usually obtained from a grow operation.

2. **Trimmer:** A device used to remove the leaves and stems from the cannabis flower.

3. **Dry Sifters:** This is a type of screen used to separate the trichomes from the flower.

4. **CO2/Ethanol Extractor:** This is a machine used to extract the cannabinoids from the plant material using a safe and efficient process.

5. **Rotovap Machine:** This machine is used to concentrate and evaporate the cannabis extract.

6. **Vacuum Oven:** A specialized oven used to evaporate solvents from the extract.

7. **Glassware:** This includes beakers, flasks and other glass labware used in the extraction process.

8. **Solvents:** Solvents used in cannabis extraction include butane, ethanol and CO2.

9. **Vacuum Chamber:** A vacuum chamber is used to remove the solvent from the extract.

10. **Lab Equipment:** Lab equipment such as a hot plate, syringe filter, and a magnetic stirrer bar are essential tools for cannabis extraction.

11. **Precision Scale:** A precision scale that can measure down to the milligram is essential for accurate dosing of cannabis extracts.

12. **Vacuum Pump:** A vacuum pump is used to remove gasses from the extraction vessel, making it safe to use.

It's important to note that the tools and materials used for cannabis extraction can vary depending on the process and the desired outcome of the product. Furthermore, cannabis extraction is a highly regulated industry, and the safety of the final product depends on the use of safe and efficient techniques. A thorough understanding of the process and the chemicals and equipment used is necessary to produce a safe, effective, and enjoyable product.

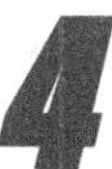

TYPES OF CANNABIS EXTRACTS

The process for making each type of cannabis extract can be complex and require specialized equipment and techniques. Here is a brief overview of how some common types of cannabis extracts are made:

1. **Dabs:** Dabs are typically made by using a process called butane extraction, which involves using butane gas to extract the cannabinoids from the dried cannabis flower. The resulting extract is then placed in a vacuum chamber to remove any residual butane, resulting in a high-potency concentrate.

2. **Hash:** Hash is produced by collecting the trichomes and resin glands from the dried and cured cannabis flower using specialized sifting or screening techniques. The trichomes are then pressed together to create a hashish cake, which can be further processed to create different types of hash.

3. **Kief:** Kief is typically made by using a specialized sifting or screening box to collect the trichomes and resin glands from the dried and cured cannabis flower. The resulting kief is then pressed together to create a hashish cake or used as a topping for bowls or joints.

4. **Rosin:** Rosin is produced by pressing dried and cured cannabis flower or hash between heated plates to extract the cannabinoids and terpenes. The resulting extract is then collected and scraped off the plates, resulting in a light yellow, wax like substance.

5. **Butter:** is made by infusing clarified butter with dried and cured cannabis flower or hash using either a stovetop or slow cooker method. Once cooled, the butter can be used to cook, bake, or mix into drinks.

6. **Tinctures:** Tinctures are typically made by simmering dried and cured cannabis flower in a high-proof alcohol, such as vodka, for an extended period of time. The resulting solution is then strained and bottled for use.

7. **Hash Oil:** Hash oil, also known as hashish oil or hashish wax, is a concentrated cannabis extract that is typically made by extracting the trichomes and terpenes from the cannabis plant using a solvent such as butane, propane, or CO2. The remaining material is then filtered, and the resulting oil is often refined to create a more stable and potent product.

It's important to note that each of these processes requires careful attention to detail, high-quality starting material, and a thorough understanding of the science behind cannabis extraction.

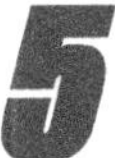

HOW TO MAKE CANNABUTTER

Cannabutter is an easy method for extracting the active substances of hemp plants, which will make them easier to digest. To learn how to make cannabutter for the first time, this is a step by step guide:

1. **Gather your supplies:** You'll need a source of cannabis, usually in the form of flower, trim, or shake. You'll also need a crockpot or double-boiler, a strainer or metal mesh sieve, a spatula, and some unsalted butter.

2. **Decarboxylation:** The first step is to decarboxylate the cannabis before infusing it into the butter. To do this, place the flower, trim or shake on a baking tray and bake in the oven at 250°F (120°C) for around 25-30 minutes. This activates the THC and CBD in the cannabis.

3. **Infuse the butter:** Melt the unsalted butter in a crockpot or double-boiler. Once melted, add the decarboxylated cannabis and allow it to simmer for around 2-3 hours on low heat. Stir occasionally to ensure even distribution of the cannabis.

4. **Strain the butter:** Strain the mixture through a strainer or mesh sieve to remove any flower or plant material.

Be sure to press down on the plant material to extract as much of the cannabinoid-rich butter as possible.

5. **Store the butter:** The strained butter can be stored in an airtight container in the refrigerator or freezer. It's important to use butter, as it has a higher fat content than other spreading butters, so the cannabinoids can bind more easily to the fat molecules.

It's important to note that the strength of the butter will depend on the amount and potency of the cannabis used. Start with a low dosage around 10-2

Once you've consumed the edible, it could take up to an hour to feel the effects. The length of time it takes to kick in can vary based on your metabolism, tolerance level, and the other substances in your system. It is important to start low and go slow when it comes to cannabis edibles. It's not uncommon for edibles to feel like they're not working, and then all of a sudden they hit. It's important to have patience and give it time to kick in, and always start with a low dose to feel out your tolerance level.

Enjoy! Now that the edibles have kicked in, it's time to enjoy the ride! Relax, put on some music or a movie, and enjoy the experience. It's important to always listen to your body and mind and adjust your actions accordingly. Remember, the most important thing is safety and a good time.

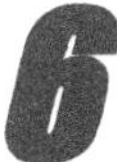

HOW TO MAKE CANNABUTTER-INFUSED EDIBLES

A few more ingredients are needed to make weed infused edibles, but the process is still manageable. How to make cannabutter infused edibles for the first time, see this step by step guide:

1. Gather your supplies: You'll need a source of cannabis, usually in the form of flower, trim, or shake. You'll also need a crockpot or double-boiler, a strainer or metal mesh sieve, a spatula, unsalted butter, a baking tray, a mixing bowl, cookie or cupcake liners, and some ingredients to make weed-infused edibles.

2. Decarboxylation: The first step is to decarboxylate the cannabis before infusing it into the butter. To do this, place the flower, trim or shake on a baking tray and bake in the oven at 250°F (120°C) for around 25-30 minutes. This activates the THC and CBD in the cannabis.

3. Make cannabutter: Melt the unsalted butter in a crockpot or double-boiler. Once melted, add the decarboxylated cannabis and allow it to simmer for around 2-3 hours on low heat. Stir occasionally to ensure even distribution of the cannabis.

4. Strain the butter: Strain the mixture through a strainer or mesh sieve to remove any flower or plant material. Be sure to press down on the plant material to extract as much of the cannabinoid-rich butter as possible.

5. Use the cannabutter: Use the cannabutter in place of regular butter in your preferred edible recipe. You can use it to make cookies, brownies, cakes, or other treats. When baking, be sure to preheat your oven to the recommended temperature and bake for the recommended time.

6. Infuse the ingredients: Before using the cannabutter, you may need to infuse it into the other ingredients (like sugar or flour) for optimal potency. To do this, melt the appropriate amount of cannabutter and mix it with the sugar or flour until thoroughly combined. This will ensure that the cannabutter is evenly distributed throughout the edible.

7. Bake the edibles: Preheat your oven to the recommended temperature and follow the recipe instructions for baking. Be sure to check on the edibles regularly and remove them from the oven when they're done baking.

Enjoy. Now that the edibles are baked, it's time to enjoy the results of your hard work! Sit back, relax and enjoy the experience. Be aware that edibles can take longer than the other methods of consumption to feel the effects, and the effects can last longer. Always start with a small dose and wait at least one hour before consuming any more. It's best to be in a safe, comfortable environment with familiar people in case you need something to ease the high.

7

HOW TO MAKE TOPICALS AND SALVES

Making topical products like balms, creams, and salves is a great way to use your cannabis without inhaling it. Here's a step-by-step guide on how to make your own topical cannabis products:

1. Gather your supplies: You'll need a source of cannabis (usually in the form of flower, trim, or shake), a cooking pan, a double-boiler, a strainer or metal mesh sieve, a spatula, a jar or container, unprocessed organic coconut oil or shea butter, and essential oils (optional).

2. Decarboxylation: The first step is to decarboxylate the cannabis before infusing it into the oil. To do this, place the flower, trim, or shake on a baking tray and bake in the oven at 250°F (120°C) for around 25-30 minutes. This activates the THC and CBD in the cannabis.

3. Infuse the oil: Melt the unprocessed coconut oil or shea butter in a double-boiler or a pan. Once melted, add the decarboxylated cannabis and allow it to simmer for around 2-3 hours on low heat. Stir occasionally to ensure even distribution of the cannabis.

4. Strain the oil: Strain the mixture through a strainer or mesh sieve to remove any flower or plant material. Be sure to press down on the plant material to extract as much of the cannabinoid-rich oil as possible.

5. Optional: Add essential oils to the infused oil. These can add scent, flavor, and medicinal benefits to the topical, depending on the type of oil you use. Some examples of essential oils are grapefruit, lavender, and peppermint.

6. Apply: Once the oil has cooled down, apply it to your skin. You can use a carrier oil (like jojoba or almond oil) if you prefer a lighter consistency. It's important to test a small amount of the oil on a small patch of skin before applying it to a larger area.

7. Use as needed: Use the topical daily to alleviate pain, inflammation, and other ailments. You can also try using it before going to bed or after exercising to promote relaxation and rest.

It's important to note that homemade topical products will contain trace amounts of THC, and they are not as potent as other cannabis products like edibles or vapes. Therefore, they will not produce a psychoactive effect similar to other cannabis products. However, some users report feeling a mild relaxation after using topicals. It's also important to keep the products away from children and pets, as even trace amounts of THC can affect them.

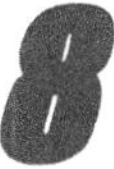

HOW TO MAKE TINCTURES

Making cannabis tinctures is one of the easiest ways to extract the medicinal benefits of cannabis without smoking or vaping it. Here's a step-by-step guide on how to make cannabis tinctures:

1. **Gather your supplies:** You'll need a source of cannabis (usually in the form of flower, trim, or shake) and a high-proof alcohol (like everclear or vodka). You can also use vinegar if you prefer a non-alcoholic tincture.

2. **Decarboxetine:** Decarboxylating the cannabis is an important step, as it activates the THC-A into THC. To do this, place the flower, trim, or shake on a baking tray and bake in the oven at 250°F (120°C) for around 25-30 minutes. This activates the THC and CBD in the cannabis.

3. **Infuse:** Add the cannabis to a glass jar along with the alcohol (or vinegar) and shake well. Let the mixture steep for at least 30 minutes or up to 24 hours in a dark or cool place. Shake every few hours to ensure even distribution of the cannabis.

4. **Strain:** After the infusion period, strain the mixture through a cheesecloth or mesh sieve to remove any plant

material. Be sure to press down on the plant material to extract as much of the cannabinoid-rich alcohol as possible.

5. **Dosage:** The tincture is ready to use. Be sure to start with a low dose and gradually increase to find your effective dose. You can add the tincture to food or drinks or use it sublingually by placing it under your tongue for around 30 seconds before swallowing.

6. **Storage:** Store the tincture in a cool, dark place away from children and pets.

Tinctures offer a quick and easy way to consume cannabis without smoking or vaping. The benefits can be felt within minutes and the effects can last up to 8 hours, depending on the dose and your tolerance level. Tinctures are also more discreet than smoking or vaping, which can be convenient for those who prefer to use cannabis discreetly.

Remember: Always be mindful of your consumption and start with low doses to find your effective dose. It's important to use cannabis responsibly and know your sources.

Also remember to stay hydrated and be mindful of the environment you're in when consuming edibles. It's always important to have a safe and relaxed environment and to be responsible when consuming cannabis. Also, please do not drive or operate heavy machinery while under the influence of cannabis.

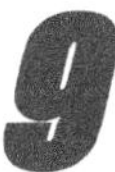

HOW TO MAKE HASH

Making hash is a fun and exciting process that can be done at home with a few ingredients. Here's a step-by-step guide on how to make hash:

1. **Gather your supplies:** You'll need cannabis (usually in the form of flower or trim) and a mesh screen or sifter to create kief, as well as wax paper or parchment paper and an empty glass container (like a jar or vial).

2. **Create kief:** To make kief, first break up the cannabis into small pieces and place them on a mesh screen or sifter. Shake the screen or sifter over a collection container to catch the keif. You can use a small brush to scrape the kief off the mesh and into the container.

3. **Freeze:** Place the keif-filled container in the freezer for at least 30 minutes, or up to an hour. This will help the trichomes (the source of the cannabinoids) to become brittle and fall off the flower more easily.

4. **Shake:** After the freezer, remove the container from the freezer and place it in a dark or cooled down place. Use a clean brush to shake the keif off the frozen flower.

5. **Press:** Place a piece of wax paper or parchment paper on a flat surface. Pack the keif into a small ball, then wrap the

paper around the ball. Press it with an empty glass container or rolling pin until it forms into a small, dense hash "coin".

6. **Store:** Store the hash in a cool, dry place away from direct sunlight.

7. **Use:** To use the hash, break off a small piece and place it on a bowl or in a joint, or sandwich it between flowers or tobacco in a cigarette. You can also break up the hash and add it to a vaporizer or dab rig.

Hash is a potent and concentrated form of cannabis that can be enjoyed in a variety of ways. It's important to start with small doses and increase slowly to find your desirable high. When using hash, always be mindful of your consumption and use cannabis responsibly.

Remember, hash-making is a personal experience that can take some practice and experimentation. Don't be afraid to try different methods and see what works best for you.

If you want to share with friends or family, be sure to let them know it's edible and that it can take a while before they feel the effects. It's always better to err on the side of caution and wait a bit longer if they are unsure how much they should eat.

Always remember to stay hydrated and be mindful of the environment you're in when consuming edibles. It's always important to have a safe and relaxed environment and to be responsible when consuming cannabis. Also, please do not drive or operate heavy machinery while under the influence of cannabis.

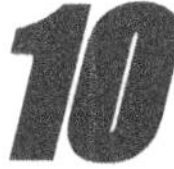

HOW TO MAKE CONCENTRATES

Making concentrates is a process of extracting the active compounds from cannabis, such as THC, CBD, and other cannabinoids. There are several techniques for making concentrates, each with its own unique advantages and disadvantages. Here's a step-by-step guide to making concentrates:

1. **Pick your method:** The first step is to choose your preferred method for making concentrates. There are many ways to make them, including solvent-based extraction, solventless extraction, and heat-press extraction. Each method has its own benefits and drawbacks, so it's important to choose the method that works best for you.

2. **Prepare your cannabis:** Before making concentrates, you need to decide what type of cannabis you'll be using. Cannabis flower is the most popular choice, but shake, trim, and kief can also be used. Make sure to break the flower into small pieces and store it in a cool, dry place before extraction.

3. **Choose your extraction method:** Solvent-based extraction uses a solvent like alcohol, butane, or CO2 to extract the active compounds from the cannabis. This

method is often the most efficient, but it can be dangerous to work with solvents and may leave residual solvents in the final product. Solventless extraction, on the other hand, uses heat or pressure to extract the active compounds without the use of solvent. This method is often more expensive but produces high-quality concentrates with less residual solvent. Heat-press extraction is a newer method that uses a combination of heat and pressure to extract the active compounds from the cannabis.

4. **Prepare your extraction setup:** Before extracting, it's important to prepare your setup. This includes having the appropriate equipment and supplies, such as a vacuum chamber, a dab rig, or a vaporizer, depending on your desired form of concentrate. You should also ensure that your work space is well-ventilated and free of any open flames or sources of ignition.

5. **Extract the cannabis:** Once your setup is prepared, you're ready to extract the cannabis. Follow the directions carefully for your chosen method of extraction. Remember to be safe when working with high pressure or solvents.
Making concentrates can be a complex and time-consuming process, but the end result is often worth it. Make sure to follow all safety guidelines and research your chosen method thoroughly before starting.

11

TIPS AND TRICKS FOR SUCCESSFUL CANNABIS EXTRACTION

Some tips and tricks to help you with successful cannabis extraction:

1. **Choose high-quality cannabis:** The first step to successful cannabis extraction is to use high-quality cannabis. Look for flowers with a high THC content, well-cured flower, and minimal plant material and seeds. Trim and shake can also be used, but they may contain less THC.

2. **Use proper extraction equipment:** The next step to successful cannabis extraction is to use proper extraction equipment. This may include a vacuum chamber, a rosin press, a butane extraction tube, or a CO_2 extraction system. Be sure to choose the right equipment for the extraction method you've chosen.

3. **Practice proper safety:** Cannabis extraction can be a dangerous process, so it's important to follow proper safety protocols. Use only proper equipment, work in a well-ventilated area, and avoid using open flames. Use gloves

and protective gear to avoid exposure to solvents or other harmful substances.

4. **Use quality solvents:** If you're using a solvent-based extraction method, it's important to use high-quality solvents. This means using solvents that are non-toxic and food-grade, such as CO_2, ethanol, or butane. Be sure to follow all instructions carefully.

5. **Monitor temperature and pressure:** In any extraction method, it's important to monitor temperature and pressure carefully. In solvent-based extraction, it's important to monitor solvent temperature during extraction to ensure it doesn't exceed the boiling point. In rosin press and CO_2 extraction methods, it's important to monitor pressure carefully.

6. **Purge your extract:** After extraction, it's important to purge the extract to remove any solvent or impurities. This can be done with a vacuum chamber or by heating the extract at low temperature.

7. **Choose the right storage method:** Once the extraction is complete, it's important to choose the right storage method. Store the extract in a cool, dark, and airtight container to prevent oxidation and degradation. Consider using glass or acrylic jars for long-term storage.

By following these tips and tricks, you can increase your chances for successful cannabis extraction. Remember, it's important to be safe, informed, and responsible when dealing with potentially dangerous materials.

Conclusion

Cannabis extraction is a scientific process that involves the removal of cannabinoids, terpenes, and other compounds from the plant material. The end result is a concentrated form of cannabis that offers a unique experience and a variety of benefits. As with any extraction process, proper safety and care during the process is essential to ensure the end product is safe and effective.

Cannabis extraction offers a wide range of methods and techniques, each with its own advantages and disadvantages. Understanding the process and choosing the right method for the desired extract consistency, purity and yield is crucial for a successful extraction. While the process can be challenging, it's also a rewarding experience that can lead to a rich and unique exploration of the cannabis plant and its many benefits.

Ultimately, cannabis extraction is a process that requires patience, precision and a willingness to experiment. The final product, whether it's an edible extract, a concentrate or a topical, is the culmination of a process that can be as rewarding as it is challenging. For those eager to explore the many possibilities offered by cannabis extraction, the journey of discovery is as rewarding as the final product itself.

There are many things to know about cannabis extracts, including the different types of extracts, the extraction methods, and their effects. It's important to understand what each type of extract is best used for, the benefits and drawbacks of each method, and the precautions to take during the extraction process. Research and education are essential for making informed decisions and ensuring a safe and enjoyable experience.

In addition to the scientific aspects, there are also cultural and traditional aspects to consider when it comes to cannabis and its extracts. The use of cannabis and its extracts can be traced back thousands of years in various cultures around the world, with different practices and traditions developed over time.

One of the most important things to remember is that cannabis and its extracts can affect each person differently, and it's important to start with a low dose and increase gradually to find the right dosage

. It's also important to choose high-quality cannabis from a trusted source, as the quality of the cannabis is reflected in the quality of the extract.

.

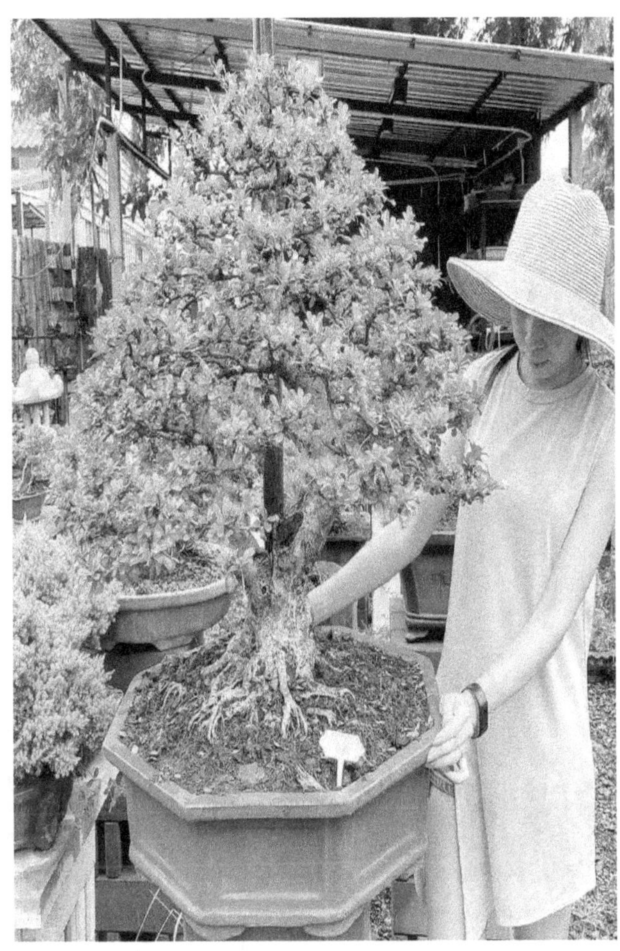

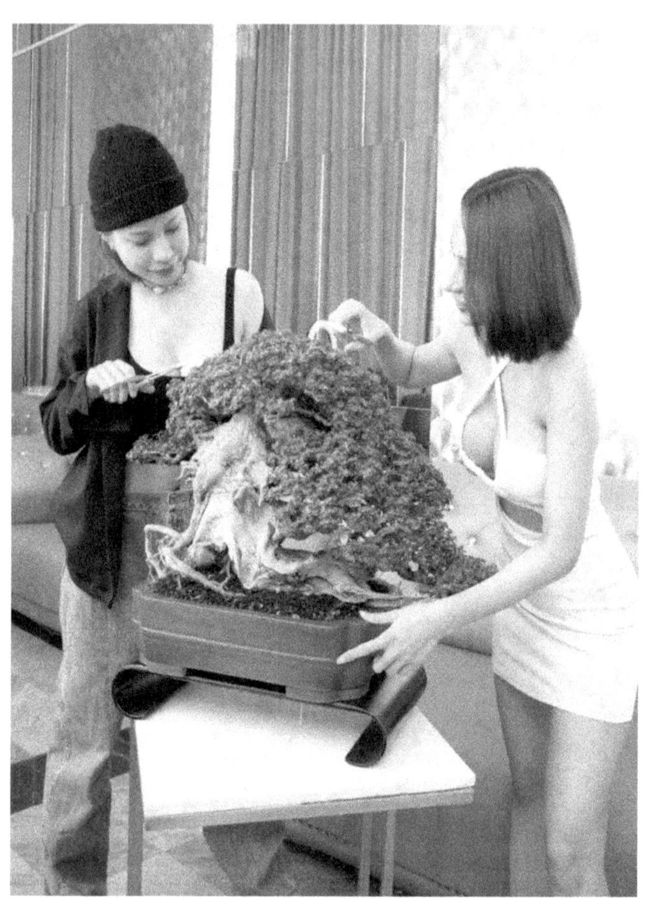